The 80/20 Rule: How Insurers Spend Your Health Insurance Premiums

SUMMARY

The Affordable Care Act holds health insurers accountable to consumers and ensures that American families receive value for their health insurance premium dollars. One such mechanism is the 80/20 rule, or Medical Loss Ratio (MLR) rule. The 80/20 rule brings consumers value, increases transparency and accountability, and promotes better business practices and competition among insurance companies.

The 80/20 rule requires insurance companies to reveal how much of premium dollars they actually spend on health care and how much on profits and administrative costs such as salaries and marketing. Now, with the implementation of the 80/20 rule, consumers can see how insurance companies spend their premium dollars and make more informed decisions when purchasing health insurance. The 80/20 rule will become even more important beginning in 2014, when consumers and small employers will have access to state-based competitive Health Insurance Marketplaces (also known as Exchanges) where individuals and small businesses can use the 80/20 information to compare the value of health insurance plans.

The 80/20 rule requires insurance companies to rebate any excess premium charged if they spend less than 80% of premiums on medical care and efforts to improve the quality of care (or at least 85% in the large group market). Under the 80/20 rule, insurance companies cannot keep more than 20% of premiums (or more than 15% in the large group market) for overhead and profits. Companies that spend 80% (85% in the large group market) or more on medical claims and improving health care quality already provide consumers with the required value for their premium dollars. In anticipation of the effective date of the 80/20 rule, some insurers have already modified their business practices and pricing to improve value to consumers for premium dollars.

The deadline for insurance companies to submit their 2011 MLR reports to the Department of Health and Human Services (HHS) was June 1, 2012.[1] HHS has analyzed these reports, and some of the key findings are:

- 66.9 million Americans are getting the required value for their health care premiums because most companies are spending at least 80% or 85% on medical claims and improving quality of care;

- 13.1 million Americans are getting rebates;

- 24.5% of health insurance companies did not meet the required MLR standard in at least one market;

---

[1] The data in this report are based on insurers' MLR reports submitted to HHS as of November 25, 2012. A few companies submitted corrected reports after determining that some of the data initially submitted was inaccurate or submitted reports after the June 1 deadline. The data in this report excludes the top and bottom 5% to eliminate outliers where appropriate.

- Rebates total approximately $1.1 billion, an average of $137 per family;

- Annual enrollee health insurance premiums in 2011 generally averaged between $1,700 and $4,700 in the individual market and between $2,400 and $5,400 for group health plans;

- Profits for companies owing rebates averaged 5.2% after payment of expenses, taxes, and rebates;

- Holding groups owing the most rebates include (in alphabetical order) Aetna, Cigna, Healthcare Service Corporation (HCSC), Humana, UnitedHealth, and WellPoint.

The 2011 80/20 rule results show important savings for consumers. These savings will continue in 2012 and beyond. Each time an issuer fails to meet the standard, rebates will be sent to enrollees. More importantly, the 80/20 rule sets a standard of transparency around plan performance, adding information about a plan's value to help inform consumers' and employers' plan choices.

KEY RESULTS FOR 2011

80/20 Rule Rebates Explained

80 million Americans are covered by health insurance plans subject to the 80/20 rule.[2] An insurer's MLR is calculated on a statewide basis, separately for the individual market, small group market, and large group market. It is not calculated for each individual or each employer group or for each plan or type of product (HMO, PPO, etc.). For example, if an insurer has health insurance business in a particular state in the individual market, small group market, and large group market, the insurer will have three separate MLRs in that state.

If an insurance company does not meet the applicable MLR standard in a particular state market, it must give rebates to all consumers within that state market in proportion to the amount of premium those consumers paid. Rebates are calculated as follows:

Rebate = (MLR standard – insurer's MLR) x (premium – taxes and fees).

The following chart (Figure 1) shows the total number of enrollees in each market, as well as the number of enrollees who will benefit from a rebate.[3]

---

[2] Some health coverage is not subject to the 80/20 rule, including employer based coverage that is self-funded, and Medicare Part C and Part D plans (Medicare plans will be subject to a separate 80/20 rule beginning 2014).

[3] The number of enrollees is estimated using life-years. Life-years are the combined number of months that have been insured during the year, divided by 12. For example, if one enrollee was only insured for the first six months of the year, and another enrollee was only insured for the last six months of the year, together this would count as one life-year.

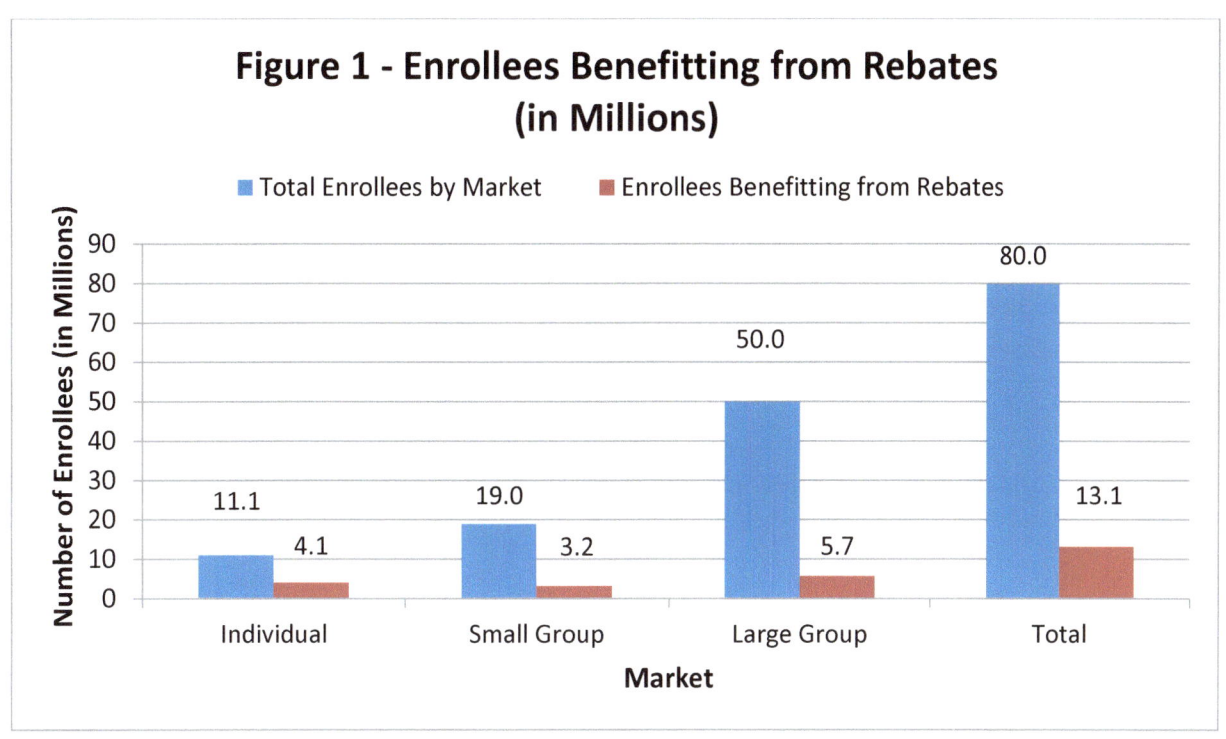

Figure 1 - Enrollees Benefitting from Rebates (in Millions)

Rebates total approximately $1.1 billion, with about $399 million in the individual market, $290 million in the small group market and $403 million in the large group market (Figure 2). While fewer companies in the large group market owe rebates (compared with the individual or small group market), the total rebate dollar amount is higher than in the individual market or the small group market. This is because companies in the large group market cover more consumers and collect more in total premiums than do the individual or small group markets.

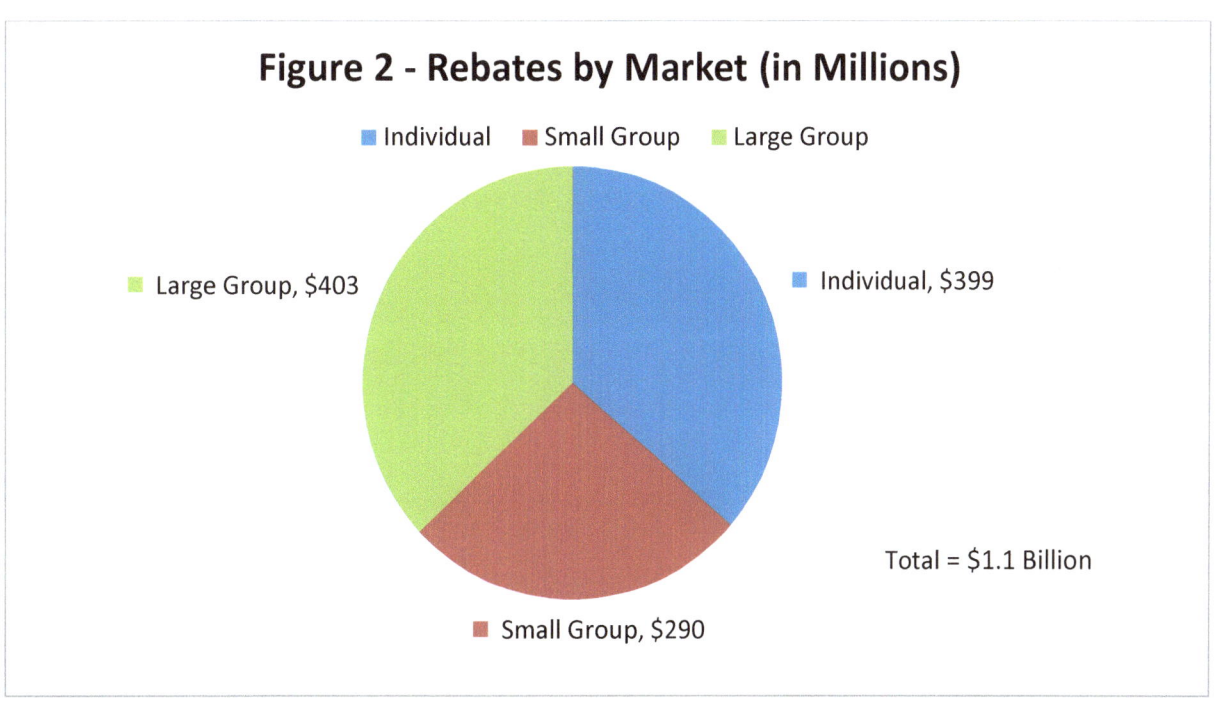

Figure 2 - Rebates by Market (in Millions)

Consumers in the individual market receive their rebate directly from the insurer, either as a cash payment or as a reduction in future premiums. For those enrolled in group health plans, where the employer is generally the policyholder, insurers do not know how much the employer and the employees each contributed to the premium. Therefore, insurers provide rebates for group health plans to employers.

Private employers are generally governed by the Employee Retirement Income Security Act (ERISA) and their handling of the rebates is regulated by the Department of Labor (DOL). DOL has issued guidance which indicates that the portion of the rebates attributable to employees' contributions to premium generally must be used for the benefit of the employees covered by the policy.[4] Self-funded plans are not subject to the MLR requirements.

Non-federal governmental employers' handling of rebates is regulated by HHS. These plans must distribute the portion of the rebate attributable to employees' contributions to premium either as a cash refund or by reducing employees' contributions to premium for the upcoming year. Because the MLR provisions require that insurers submit reports and provide rebates, and HHS does not have authority to regulate most employers, the MLR reports filed by insurers do not contain information regarding how employers are distributing the rebates.

Average Premiums

Insurers in the individual market collected more than $30 billion in total premiums in 2011, or 10% of the total reported health insurance premiums nationwide. Small group insurers received $80 billion in premiums, or 25% of the total. Large group insurers collected $209 billion in premiums, or 66% of the total premiums.

The following chart (Figure 3) shows the distribution of average annual premium per enrollee for each market. Most individual market enrollees paid annual premiums of $1,700 to $4,700 while most group market employees and their employers paid annual premiums of $2,400 to $5,400. Many factors determine annual premiums, including the benefits provided and the cost-sharing required by the insurance policy. For example, health insurance coverage with more robust benefits and lower amounts of cost-sharing for enrollees will generally have a higher premium than health insurance coverage with fewer covered benefits and higher cost sharing for enrollees.

---

[4] This Department of Labor guidance may be found at: http://www.dol.gov/ebsa/newsroom/tr11-04.html.

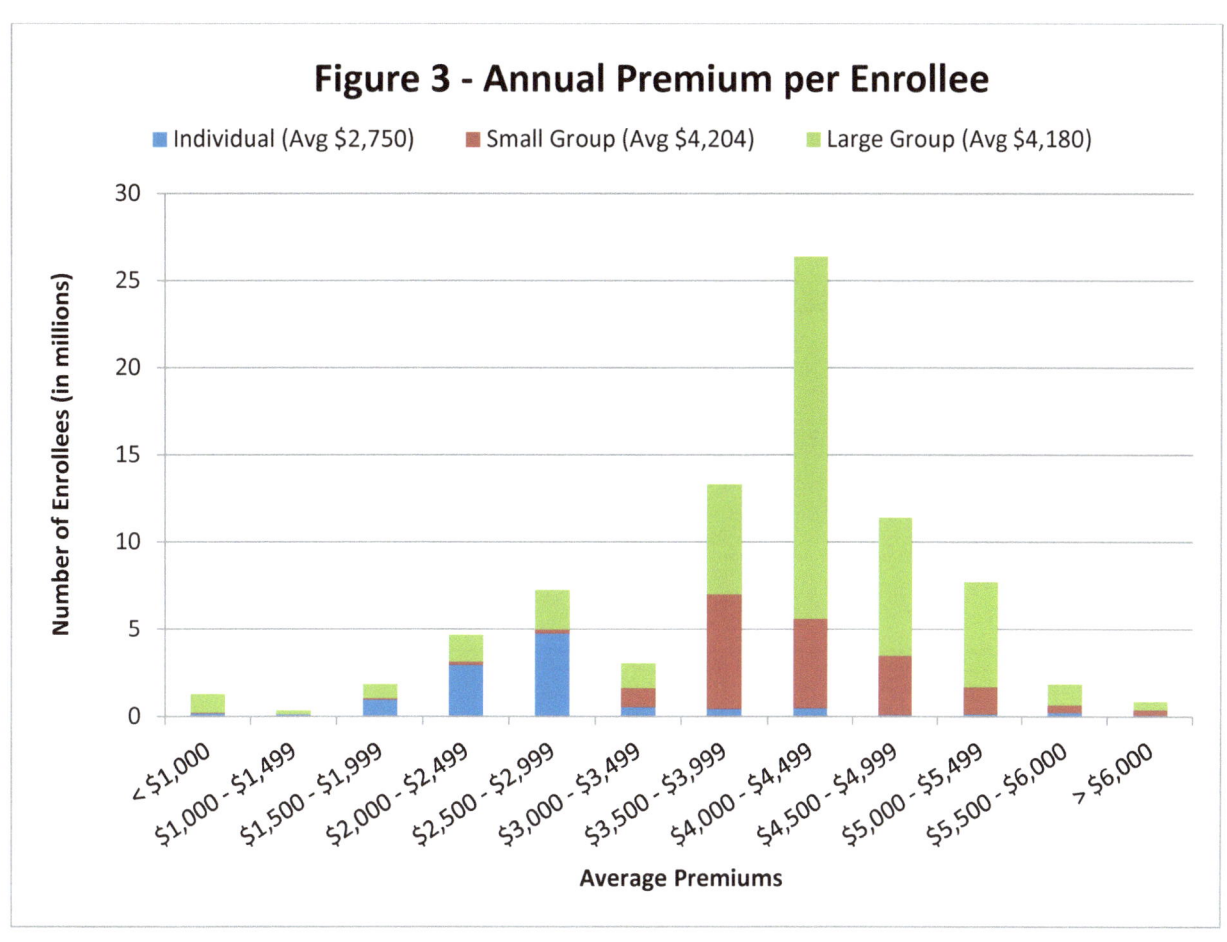

Figure 3 - Annual Premium per Enrollee

Legend: Individual (Avg $2,750) · Small Group (Avg $4,204) · Large Group (Avg $4,180)

MLR Reports Show How Insurers Spend Premiums

Insurers spend premium dollars on a variety of things, including medical care, quality improvement activities, taxes, fraud reduction activities, and administrative costs, and the remaining premium dollars become profits. The amounts spent on each activity vary widely from insurer to insurer and between markets.

The following example assumes a $2,700 individual market annual premium, with the portion of premium spent on each item based upon the average individual market spending for each category (amounts do not total exactly due to rounding).

EXAMPLE OF INSURER SPENDING:

TYPE OF COST	AMOUNT	% OF PREMIUM
Medical Claims	$2,178.90	80.7%
Activities to Improve Quality of Care	$18.90	0.7%
Allowable Fraud Reduction Expenses	$1.08	0.04%
Taxes/Fees	$67.50	2.5%
Profits and Administrative Costs	$433.62	16.1%
Total	$2,700.00	100%

The following charts (Figures 4A, 4B, and 4C) illustrate the percentage spent on each category for each market, on average.[5]

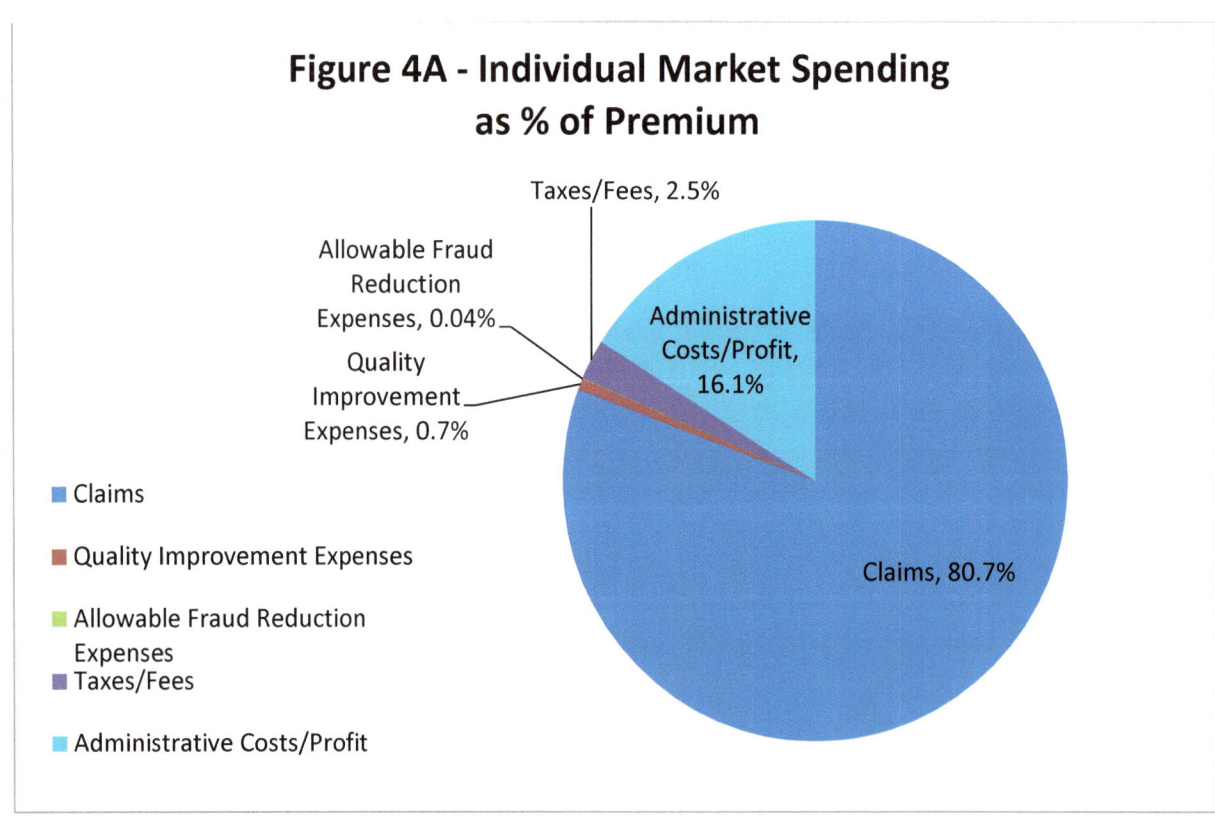

Figure 4A - Individual Market Spending as % of Premium

---

[5] The "Administrative Costs/Profits" category in Figures 4A-4C represents the difference between premium and all other expenses. It does not reflect the fact that not all issuers make expenditures on improving the quality of care or reducing fraud. It also does not reflect rebate payments and additional profits from reinsurance business. Consequently, the percentages shown in Figures 4A-4C differ slightly from those shown in Figure 6.

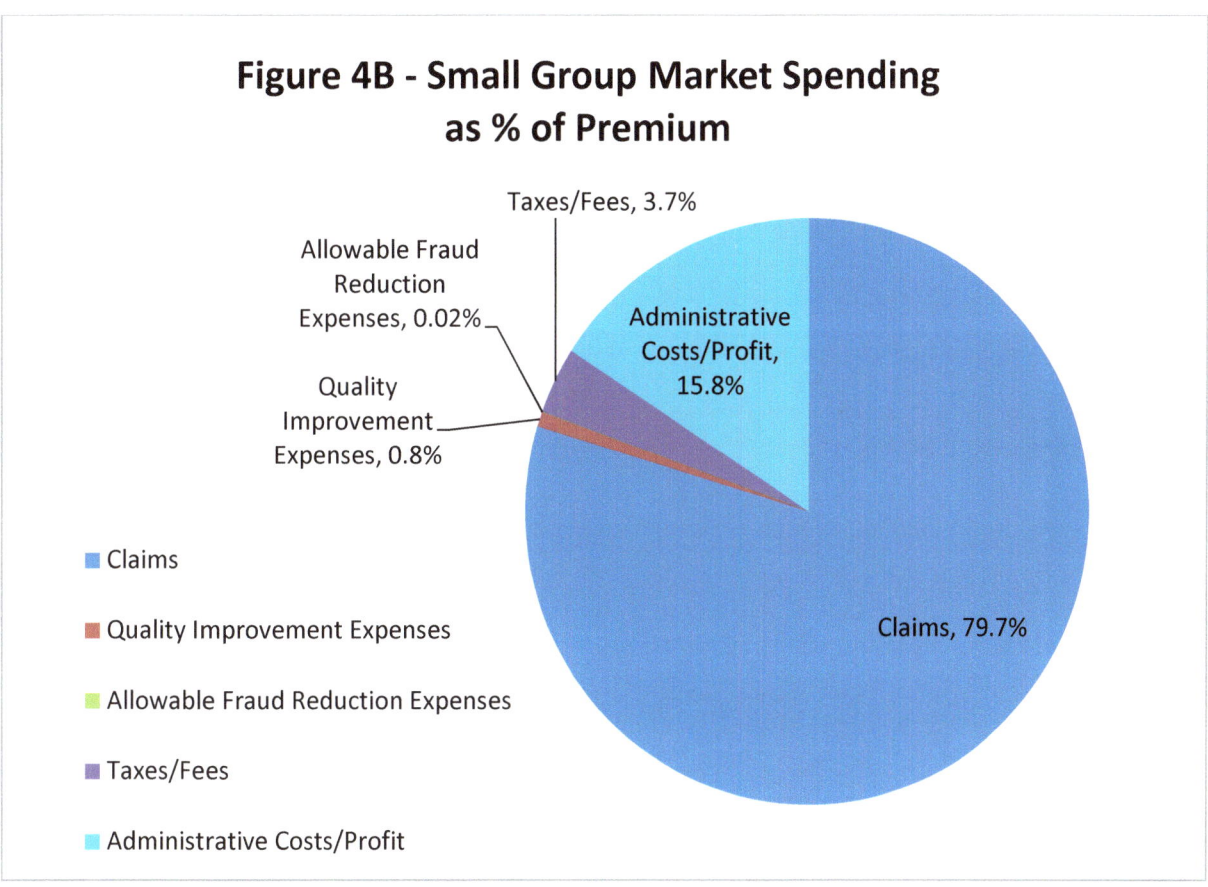

Figure 4B - Small Group Market Spending as % of Premium

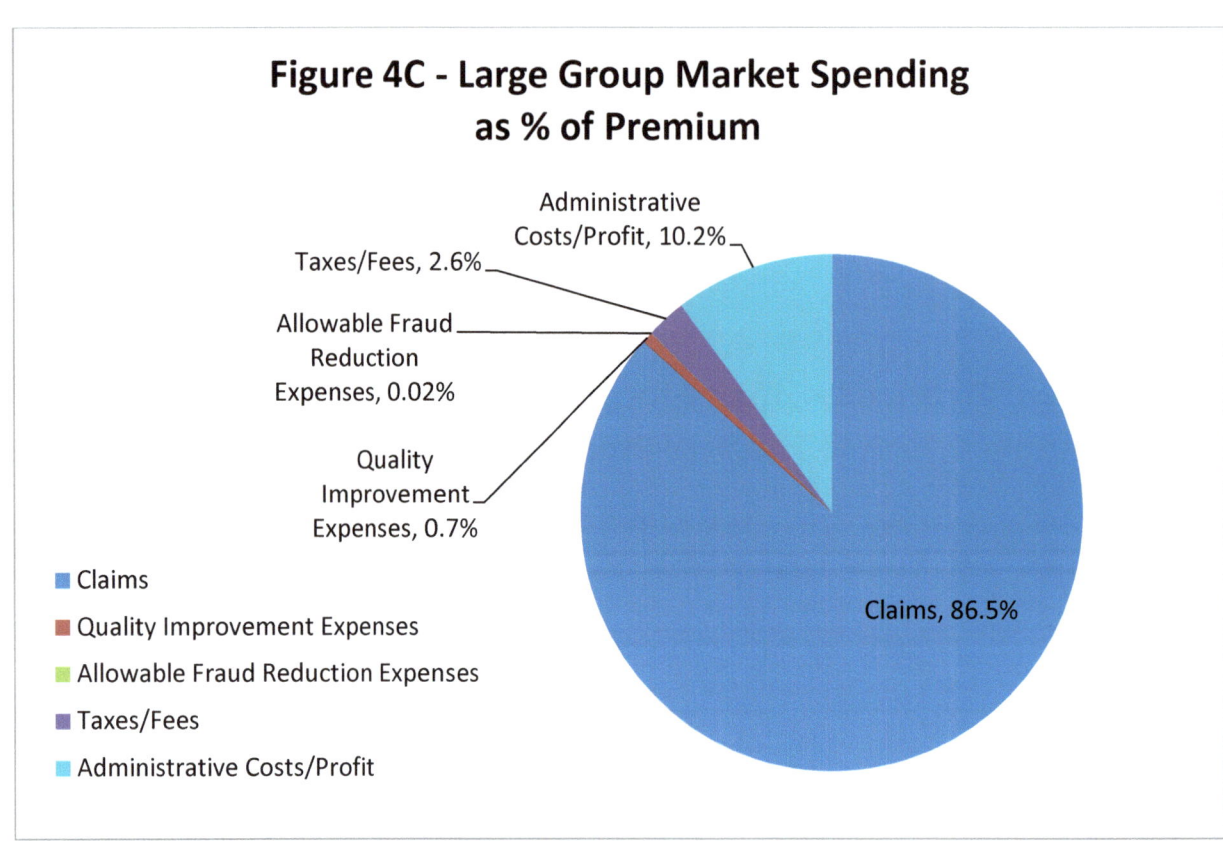

Figure 4C - Large Group Market Spending as % of Premium

- Administrative Costs/Profit, 10.2%
- Taxes/Fees, 2.6%
- Allowable Fraud Reduction Expenses, 0.02%
- Quality Improvement Expenses, 0.7%
- Claims, 86.5%

Legend:
- ■ Claims
- ■ Quality Improvement Expenses
- ■ Allowable Fraud Reduction Expenses
- ■ Taxes/Fees
- ■ Administrative Costs/Profit

Payment for Medical Care

In 2011, insurance companies spent approximately 81% of premiums on medical care in the individual market, 80% in the small group market and 87% in the large group market (Figure 5). Actual spending on medical care varied widely among insurers and state markets. Some insurers spent nothing or very little on medical care, using most of the premiums they received on administrative costs and profits, while some insurers spent more on medical care than the amount of premiums received. Spending more on medical care than premium revenue is more likely to happen if a company has a very small amount of business in a particular state market than if it has a larger amount of business.

Activities to Improve Quality of Health Care

Activities to improve the quality of health care include measurable efforts to improve health outcomes, prevent hospital readmissions, improve patient safety and reduce medical errors, and promote wellness. Sixteen percent of insurance companies reported spending nothing on improving quality of health care in 2011, while the rest generally reported spending between 0.1% and 1.4% of premium on such programs, with an average of 0.7% for companies nationwide. Insurance companies spent about the same proportion of premium on such activities in the individual, small group and large group markets (Figure 5). Collectively insurance companies spent a total of $222 million on improving quality of health care (out of $30 billion in premium) in the individual market, $610 million (out of $80 billion in premium) in the small group market, and $1.5 billion (out of $209 billion in premium) in the large group market.

Taxes

MLR and rebate calculations adjust insurers' premiums for allowable federal and state taxes, as well as licensing and regulatory fees that insurers pay to the state or federal government. The total amount paid in taxes and fees that were deducted from premium to calculate the MLR in the individual market was $748 million, or 2.5% of premium. In the small group market, insurers paid $3.0 billion or 3.7% of premium in taxes and fees. Insurers in the large group market paid $5.4 billion, or 2.6% of premium, in taxes and fees (Figure 5).

Fraud Reduction Efforts

To encourage efficient fraud reduction programs, insurers' MLRs are adjusted by the amount of fraud reduction expenses up to the amount of fraudulent claims recovered. Based on this adjustment, insurers applied to the MLR calculation $11 million of fraud reduction expenses, or 0.04% of premium, in the individual market, $15 million, or 0.02% of premium, in the small group market, and $36 million, or 0.02% of premium, in the large group market (Figure 5).

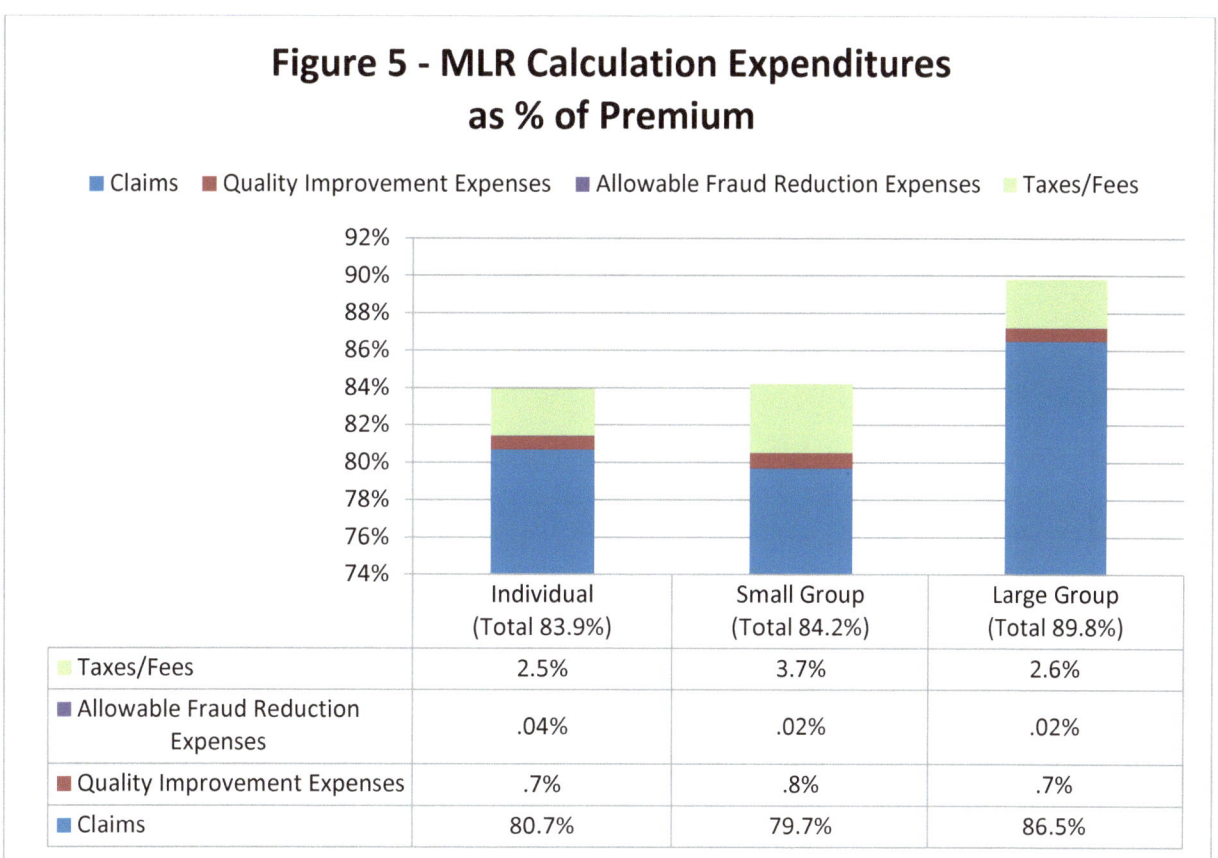

	Individual (Total 83.9%)	Small Group (Total 84.2%)	Large Group (Total 89.8%)
Taxes/Fees	2.5%	3.7%	2.6%
Allowable Fraud Reduction Expenses	.04%	.02%	.02%
Quality Improvement Expenses	.7%	.8%	.7%
Claims	80.7%	79.7%	86.5%

Administrative Costs

In 2011, health insurers collectively spent a total of $4.8 billion in the individual market, $9.6 billion in the small group market, and $15.3 billion in the large group market on administrative expenses such as marketing, salaries and bonuses. These amounts represented an average of 16% of premium in the individual market, 12% in the small group market, and 7% in the large group market, but varied widely among insurers. For example, in the individual market health insurers' total administrative costs generally ranged from 5% to 26% of premium. In the small group market, administrative costs generally ranged from 6% to nearly 19% of premium. In the large group market, administrative costs generally ranged from 4% to 12% of premium. Administrative costs as a percentage of premiums tend to be lower in the large group market since the large group market has a far greater number of enrollees, which creates economies of scale.

Profits

An insurance company's profits consist of two components: underwriting profit (the amount by which premiums exceed all expenses on medical care, quality improving activities and administration); and gains from the company's investments. In 2011, after payment of all expenses, taxes, and any MLR rebates, but before investment gains, insurance companies retained average profits of -0.4% of premium in the individual market, 5.3% in the small group market, and 3.8% in the large group market.

The following chart (Figure 6) shows insurers' average administrative costs and profits after payment of expenses, taxes and any rebates:

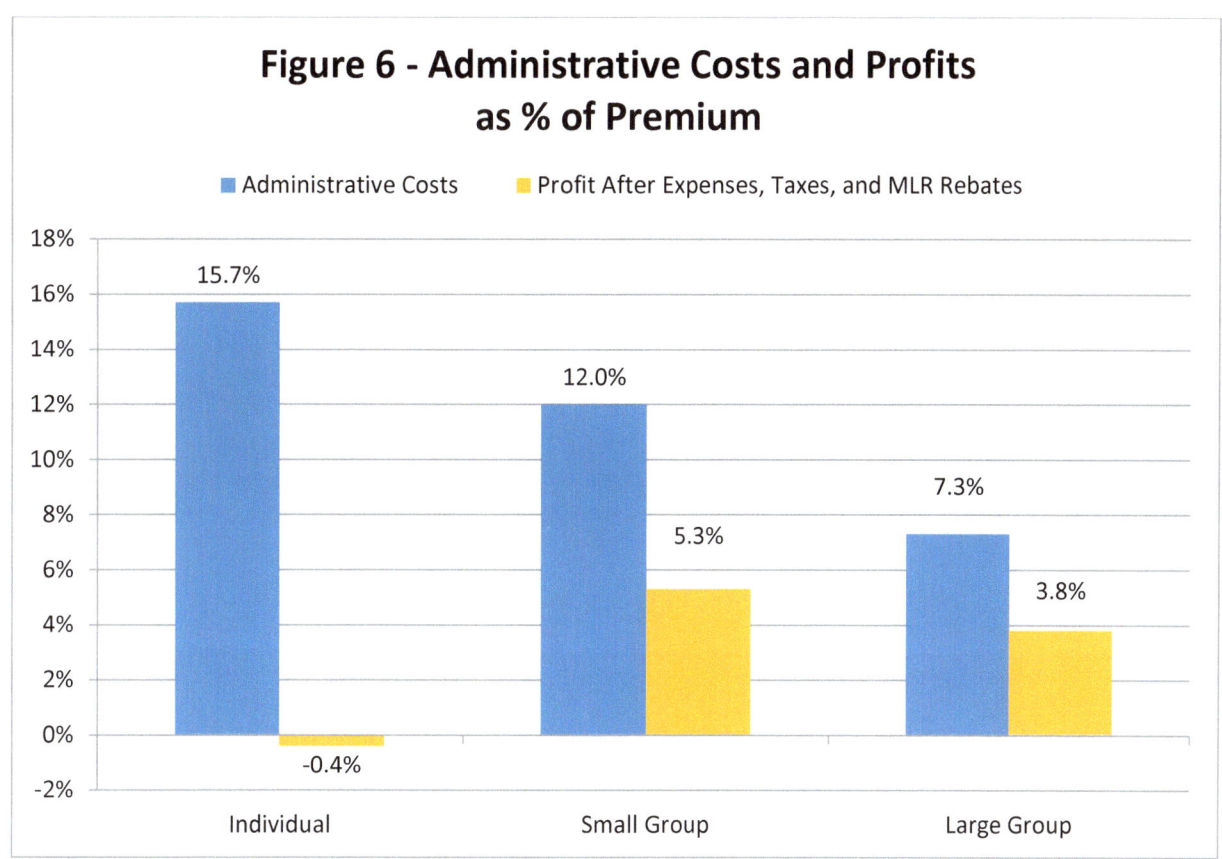

Figure 6 - Administrative Costs and Profits as % of Premium

Profits were generally lower in the individual market than in the group markets, and were lower for smaller insurers than for larger insurers. Generally, profits were significantly higher for insurers that failed to meet the MLR standard and owed rebates.

The following charts (Figures 7A, 7B, and 7C) show insurers' health insurance profit margins after payment of all expenses, taxes, and any rebates, by size of insurer:

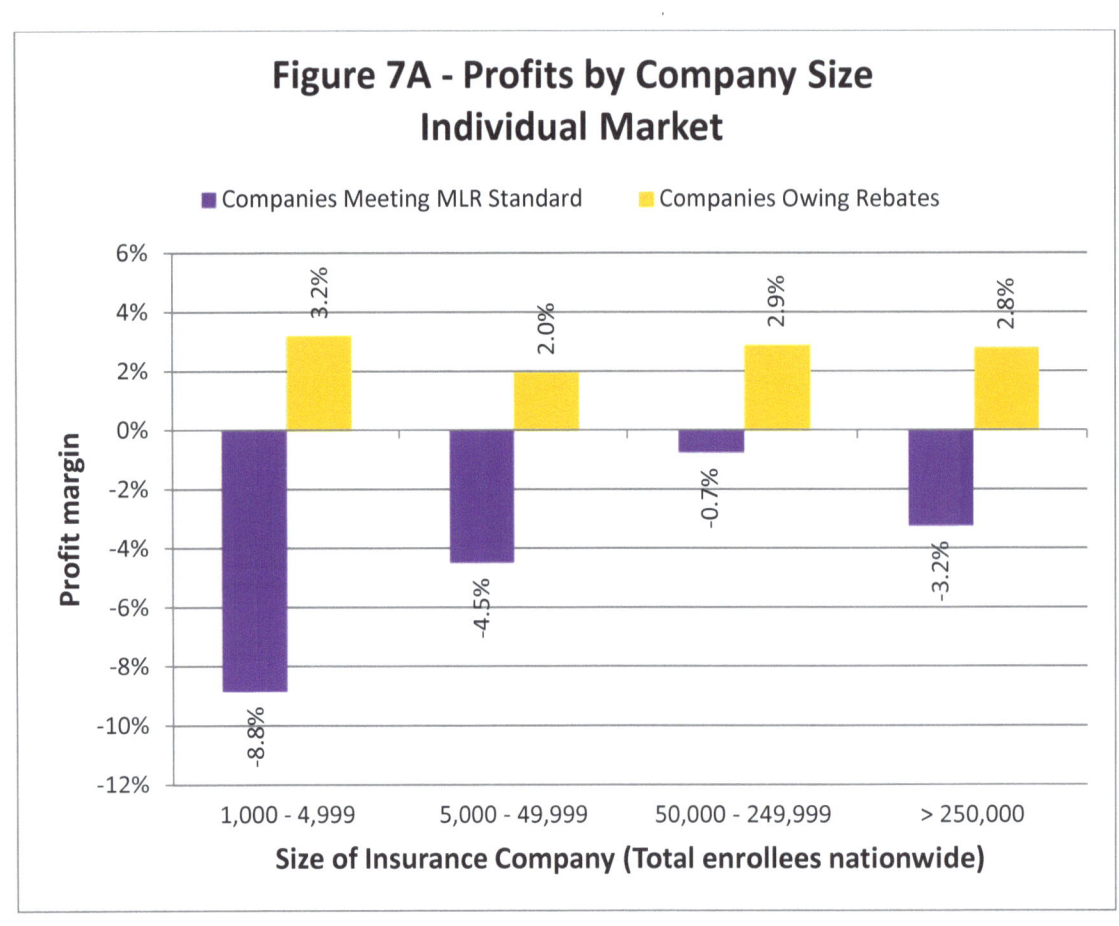

Figure 7A - Profits by Company Size Individual Market

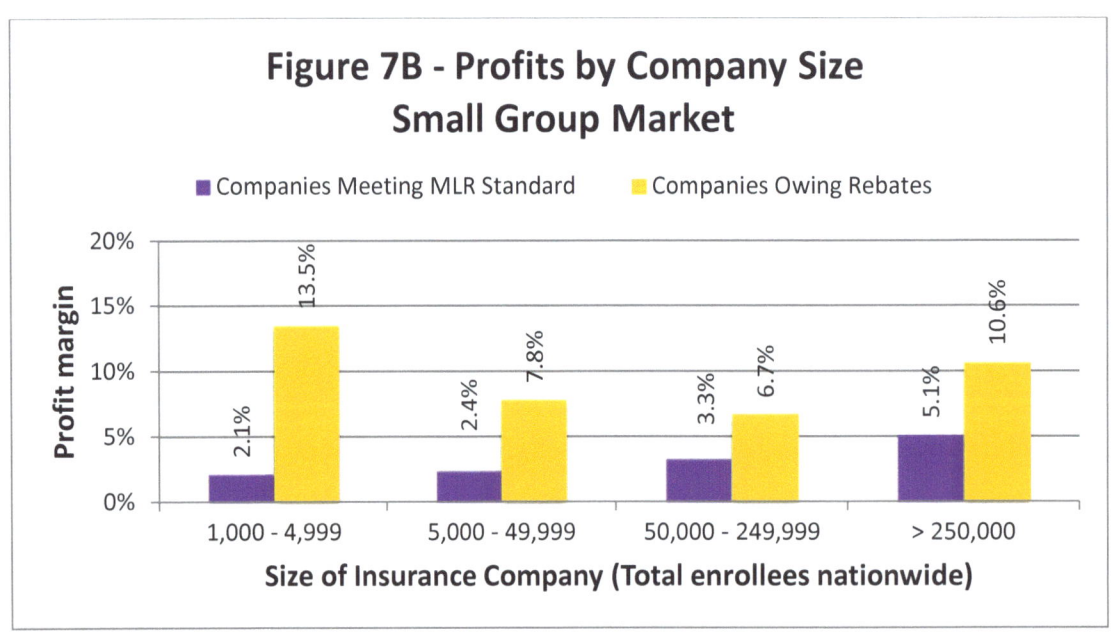

Figure 7B - Profits by Company Size Small Group Market

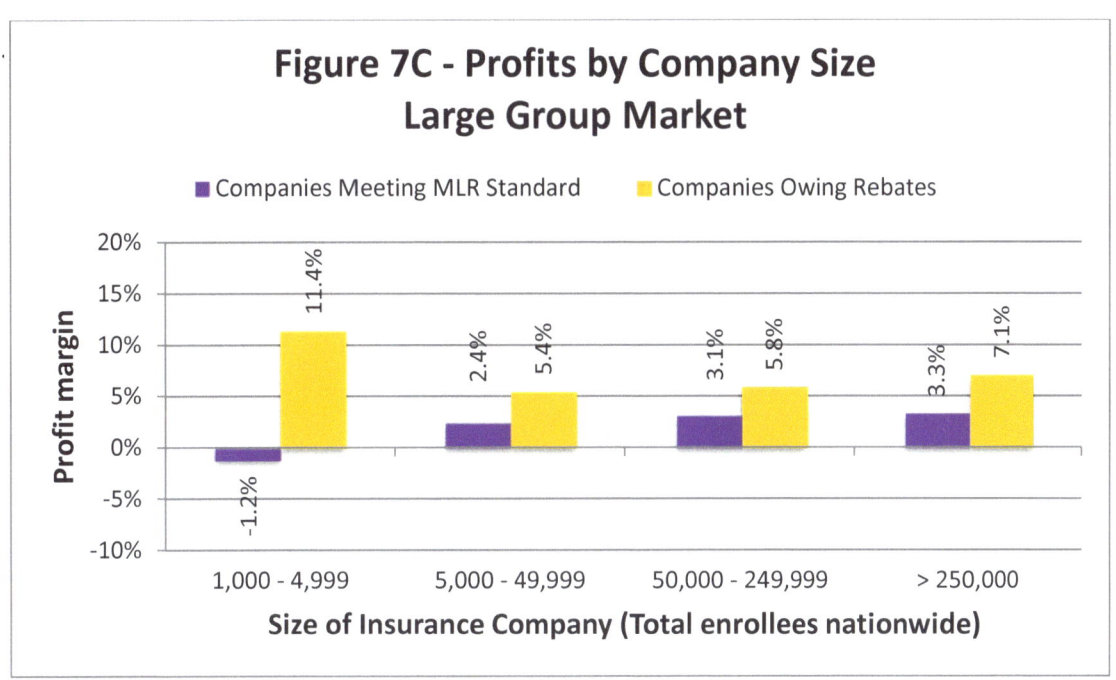

Figure 7C - Profits by Company Size
Large Group Market

■ Companies Meeting MLR Standard   ■ Companies Owing Rebates

Profit margin (y-axis): -10%, -5%, 0%, 5%, 10%, 15%, 20%

Values:
- 1,000 - 4,999: -1.2% (purple), 11.4% (yellow)
- 5,000 - 49,999: 2.4% (purple), 5.4% (yellow)
- 50,000 - 249,999: 3.1% (purple), 5.8% (yellow)
- > 250,000: 3.3% (purple), 7.1% (yellow)

Size of Insurance Company (Total enrollees nationwide)

Insurers' Rebates by Holding Group

Six insurance company holding groups, accounting for 36% of the health insurance business, owe 68% of total rebates nationwide. The total rebate payments by holding group include (in alphabetical order): Aetna ($106 million, 0.7% of earned premiums); Cigna ($77 million, 1.3% of earned premiums); Healthcare Service Corporation (HCSC) ($99 million, 0.5% of earned premiums); Humana ($74 million, 1.3% of earned premiums); UnitedHealth ($304 million, 0.8% of earned premiums); and WellPoint ($78 million, 0.2% of earned premiums) (Figure 8). All six holding groups retained profit margins of 2.7% to 8.8% after paying all taxes, expenses, and MLR rebates.

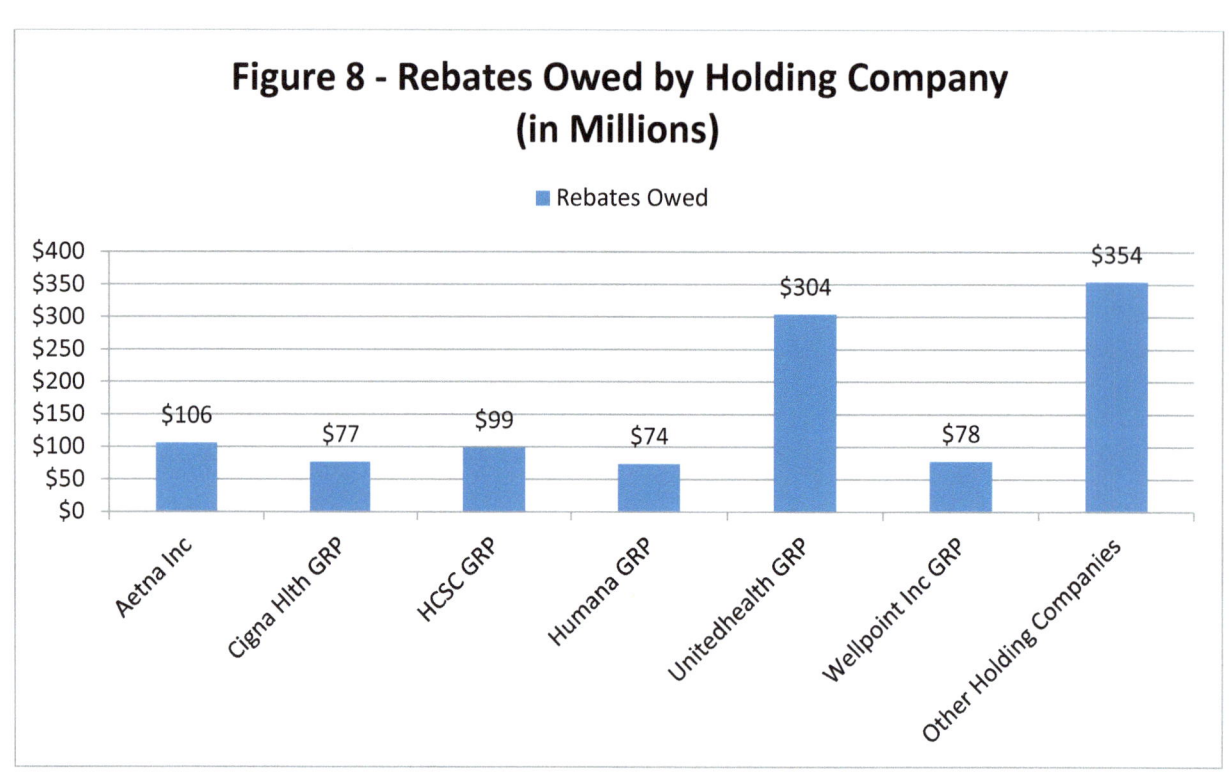

Figure 8 - Rebates Owed by Holding Company (in Millions)

Market Analyses

The average rebate differs significantly in different states and markets. The average rebate per family is $129 in the individual market, $158 in the small group market, and $134 in the large group market. Eight companies in eleven states or territories will pay an average rebate of over $1,000 per family. The actual amount of the rebate to each policyholder depends on how far a particular insurer fell below the MLR standard in a particular state market, as well as how much premium a particular policyholder paid. For example, a policyholder who paid a total of $10,000 in premiums will receive a lower rebate than a policyholder who paid a total of $15,000 in premiums if they were both in the same state market and insured by the same company.

Under the 80/20 rule, if a state establishes a higher MLR than 80% for the individual or small group market or 85% for the large group market, that higher standard is simply substituted.[6] The 80/20 rule also permits HHS to temporarily adjust the MLR standard in a state's individual market if that state shows that the 80% standard has a reasonable likelihood of destabilizing the state's individual market.[7]

---

[6] In 2011, New York generally applied an 82% standard to its individual and small group markets and Massachusetts generally applied an 88% standard to its small group market.
[7] For 2011, Georgia, Iowa, Kentucky, Maine, North Carolina, New Hampshire, and Nevada were granted adjustments. Kentucky, North Carolina, and Nevada are expected to apply the 80% MLR standard beginning in 2012.

While in most states some consumers will benefit from rebates, in a small number of states every insurance company already provided consumers with the required value for their premium dollars. No rebates will be paid to consumers in these states where every insurer met the MLR standard for that state.

As expected, the states with the largest insured population generally have the largest number of families owed rebates as well as the largest total amount of rebates: California (1.3 million insured families are owed $77.3 million in rebates); Texas (1.0 million families are owed $168.5 million); Florida (0.8 million families are owed $123.6 million); and New York (0.6 million families are owed $95.6 million). However, except for Texas, the states with the largest *proportion* of families owed a rebate are not the biggest states: District of Columbia (60% of 0.5 million insured families are owed a rebate); Arizona (59% of 0.6 million); Missouri (50% of 0.7 million); Texas (45% of 2.2 million); Oklahoma (43% of 0.4 million); and South Carolina (42% of 0.4 million). In these states, the largest insurers failed to meet the MLR standard in at least one market, which explains why a large proportion of policyholders are owed a rebate.

The following charts (Figures 9A – 9G) show the average amount of the rebate owed in the six regions of the United States and the territories, and the number of families benefitting from a rebate in each state of the regions and territories. The individual, small group and large group markets are combined.

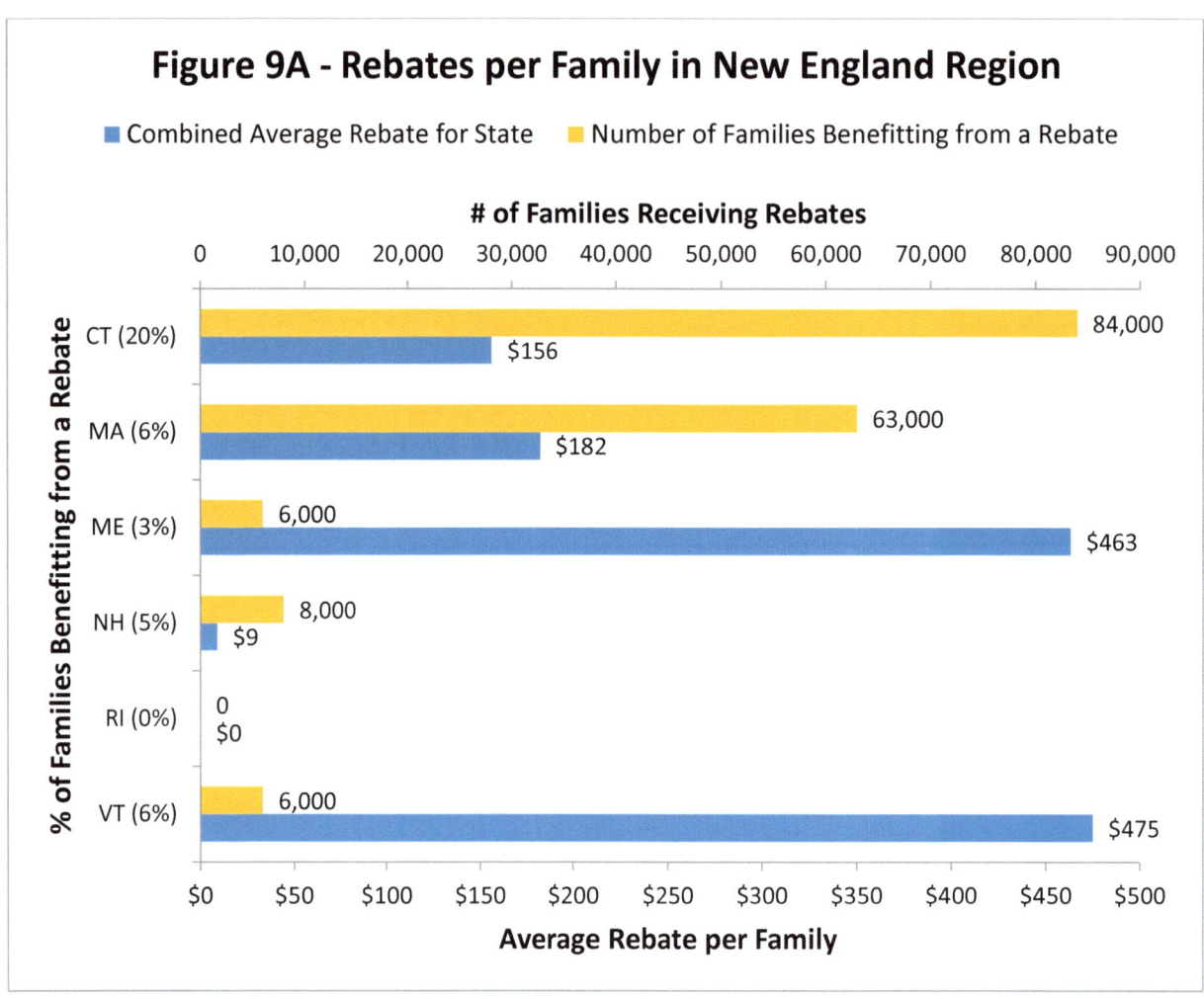

Figure 9A - Rebates per Family in New England Region

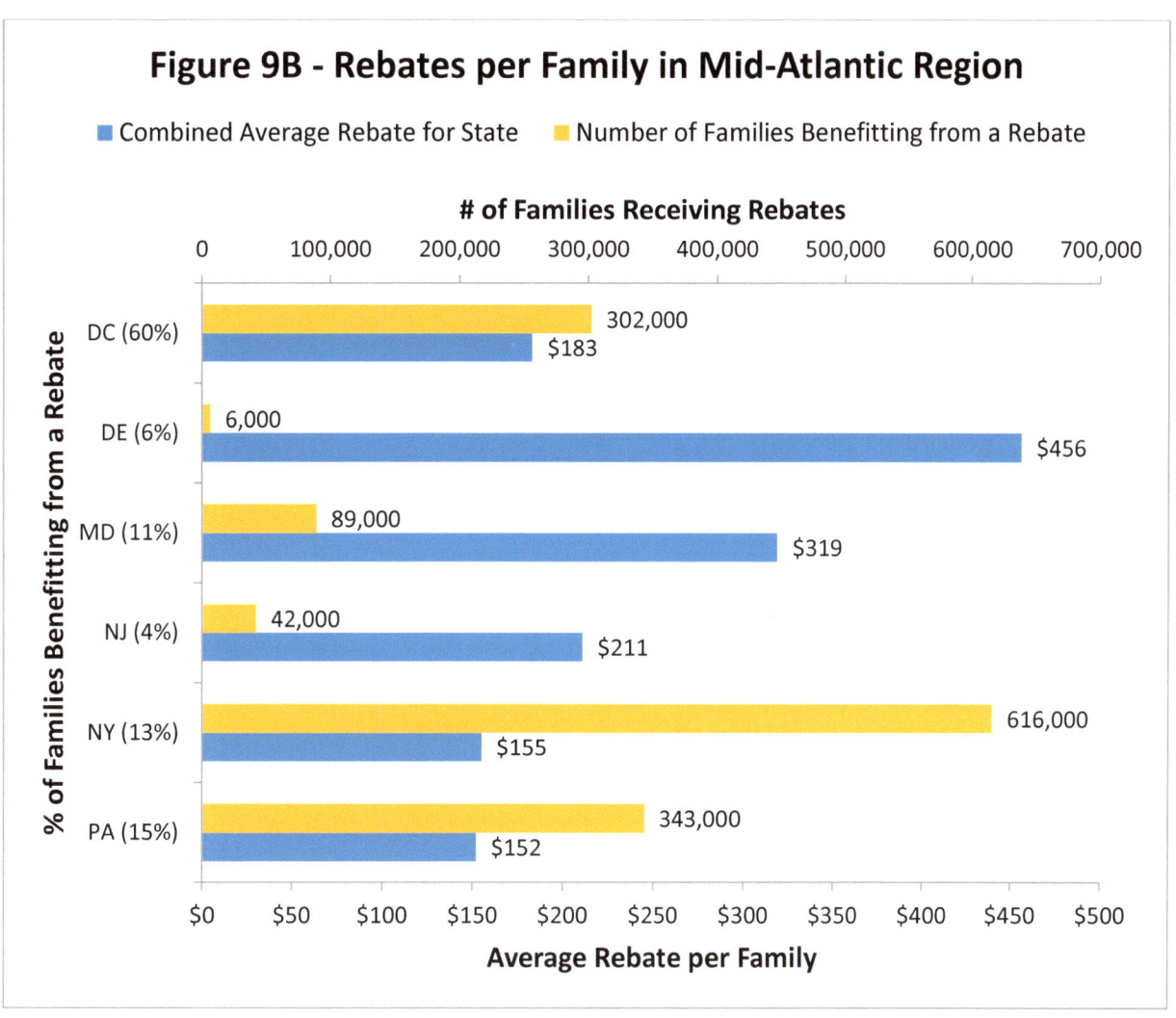

Figure 9B - Rebates per Family in Mid-Atlantic Region

■ Combined Average Rebate for State   ■ Number of Families Benefitting from a Rebate

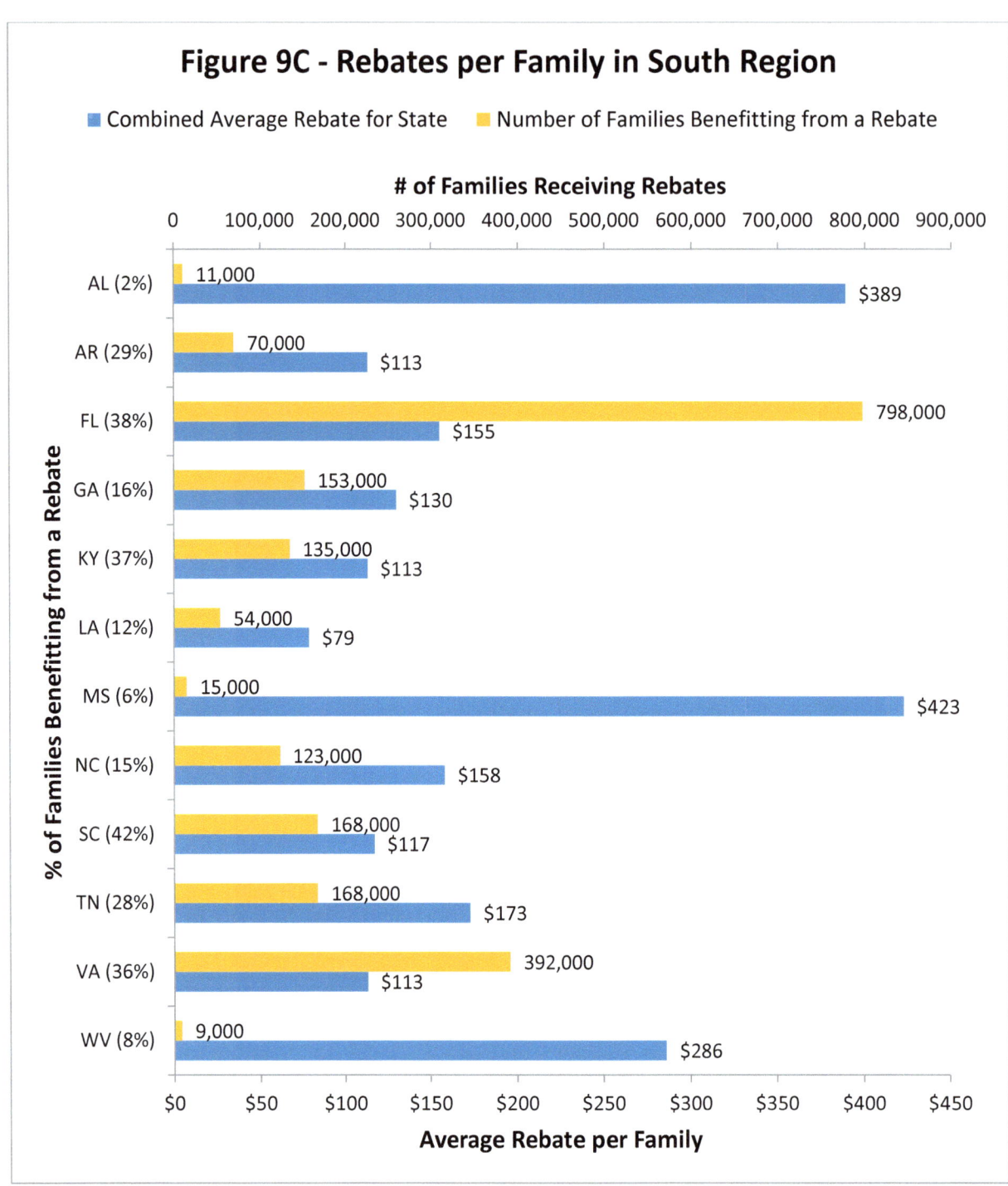

Figure 9C - Rebates per Family in South Region

■ Combined Average Rebate for State ■ Number of Families Benefitting from a Rebate

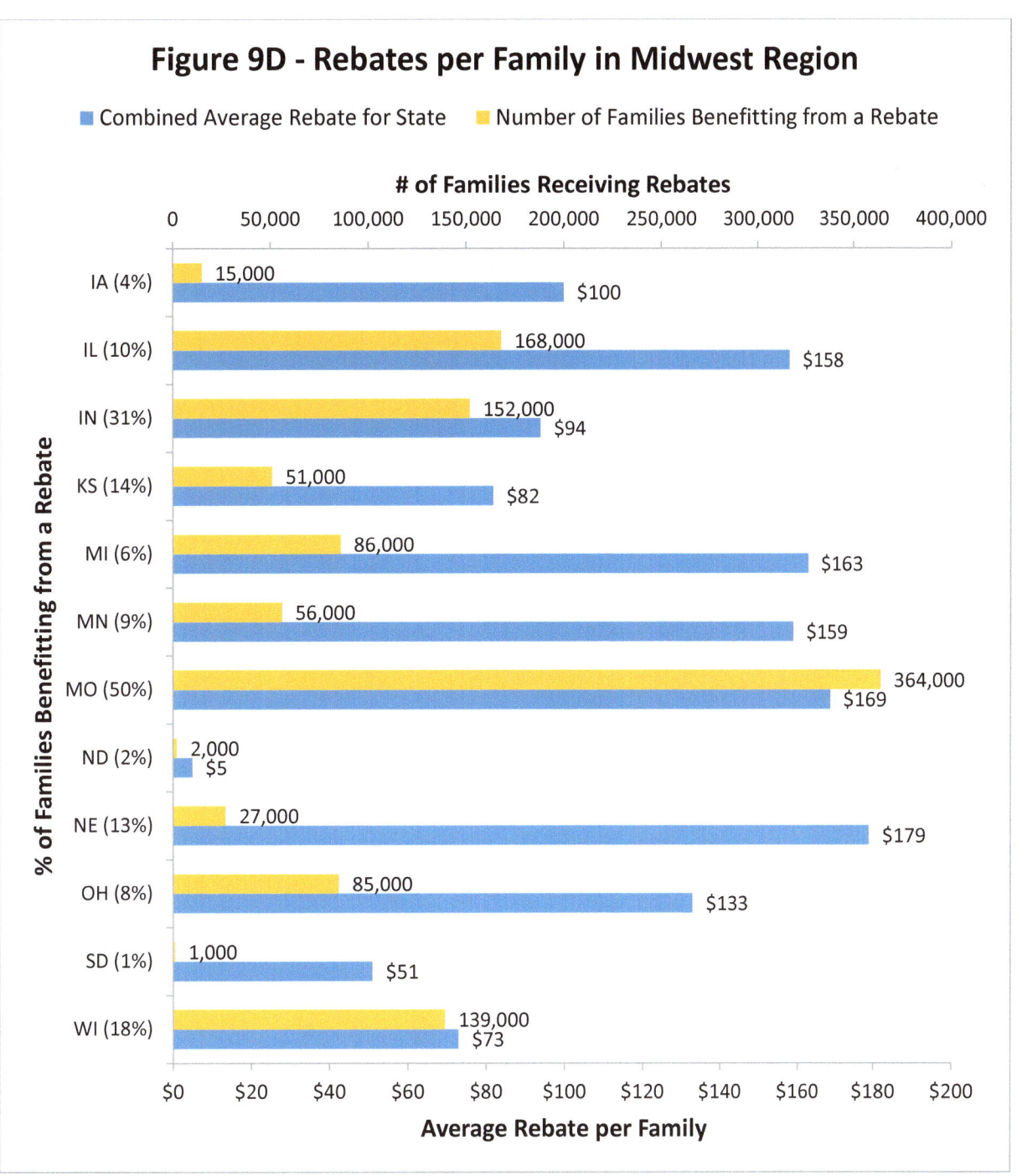

Figure 9D - Rebates per Family in Midwest Region

■ Combined Average Rebate for State ■ Number of Families Benefitting from a Rebate

# of Families Receiving Rebates

IA (4%): 15,000 / $100
IL (10%): 168,000 / $158
IN (31%): 152,000 / $94
KS (14%): 51,000 / $82
MI (6%): 86,000 / $163
MN (9%): 56,000 / $159
MO (50%): 364,000 / $169
ND (2%): 2,000 / $5
NE (13%): 27,000 / $179
OH (8%): 85,000 / $133
SD (1%): 1,000 / $51
WI (18%): 139,000 / $73

% of Families Benefitting from a Rebate

Average Rebate per Family

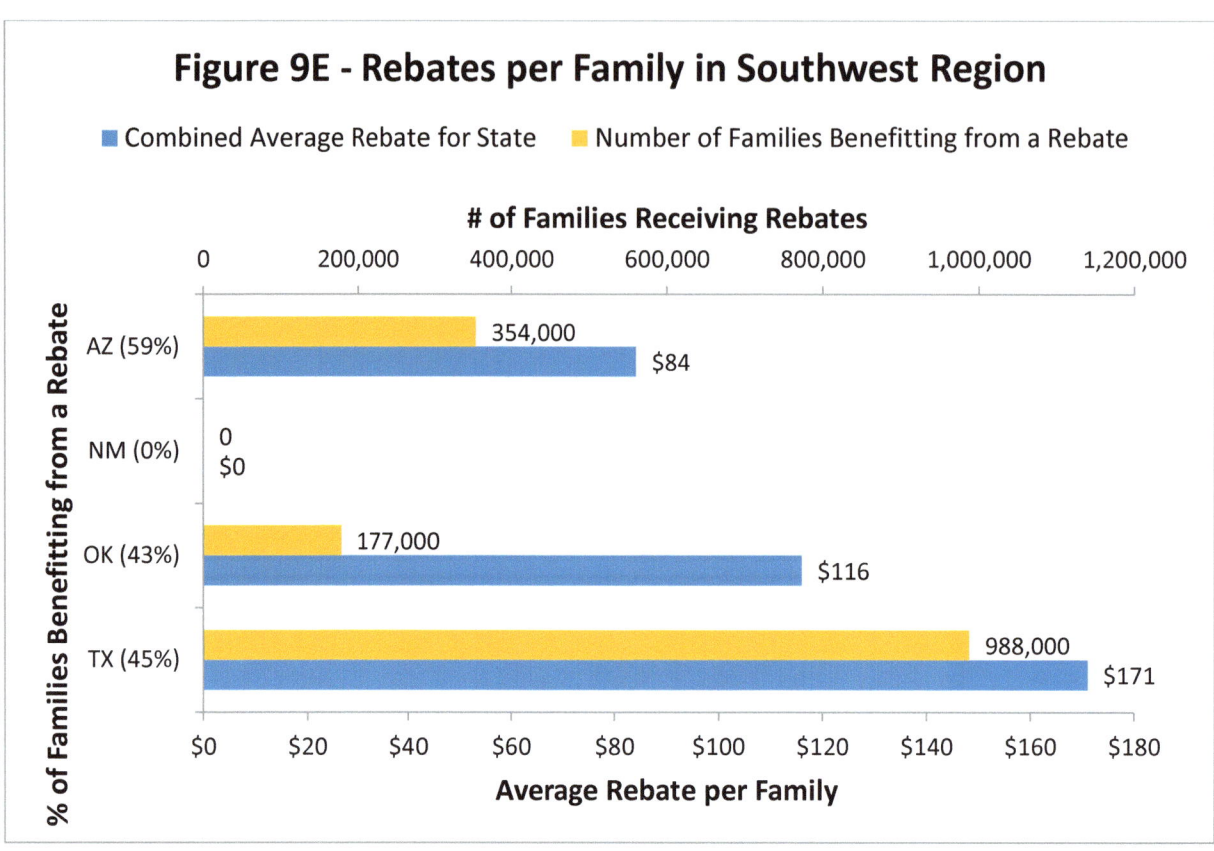

Figure 9E - Rebates per Family in Southwest Region

- Combined Average Rebate for State
- Number of Families Benefitting from a Rebate

# of Families Receiving Rebates

AZ (59%): 354,000 / $84
NM (0%): 0 / $0
OK (43%): 177,000 / $116
TX (45%): 988,000 / $171

% of Families Benefitting from a Rebate

Average Rebate per Family

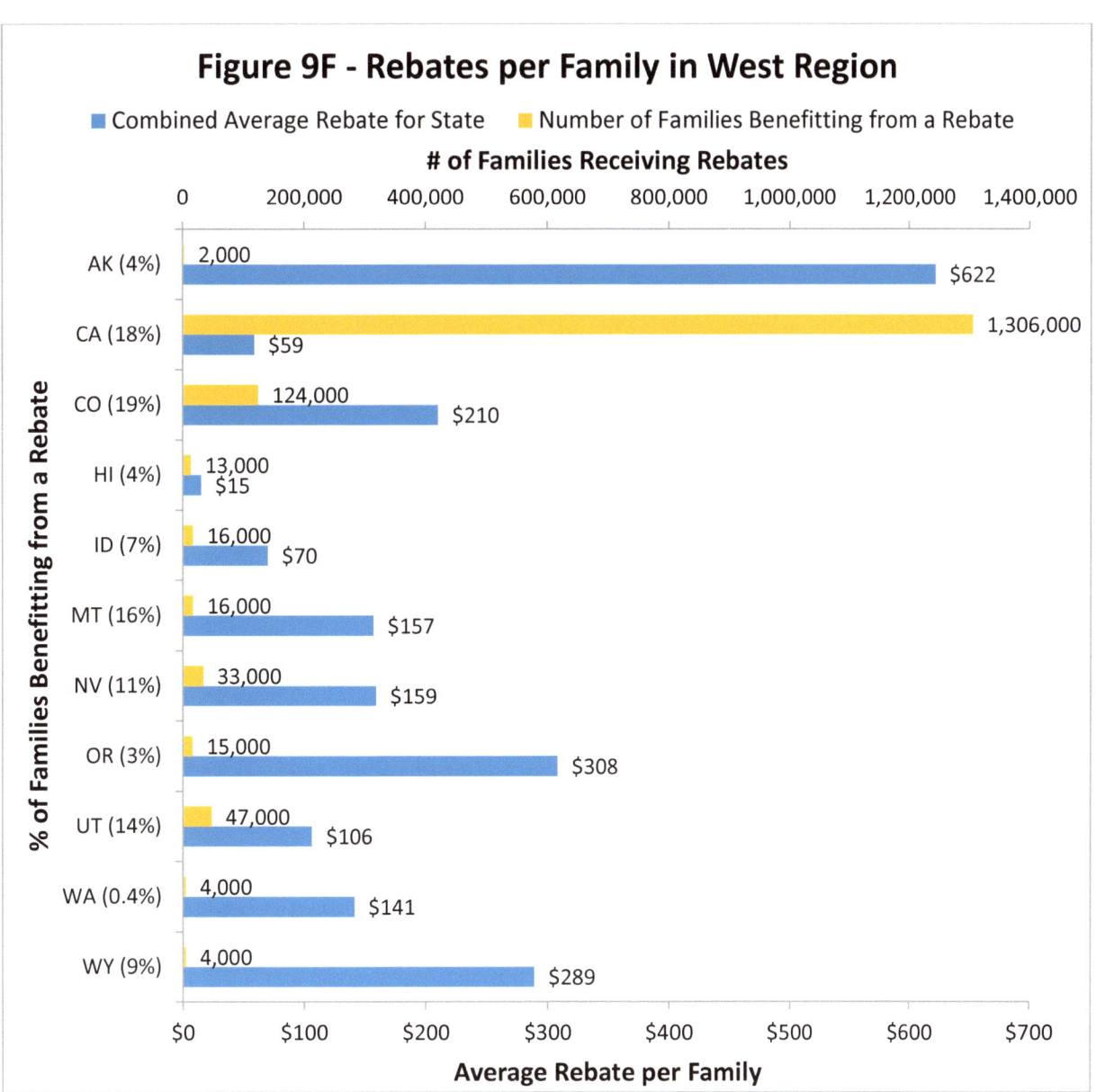

Figure 9F - Rebates per Family in West Region

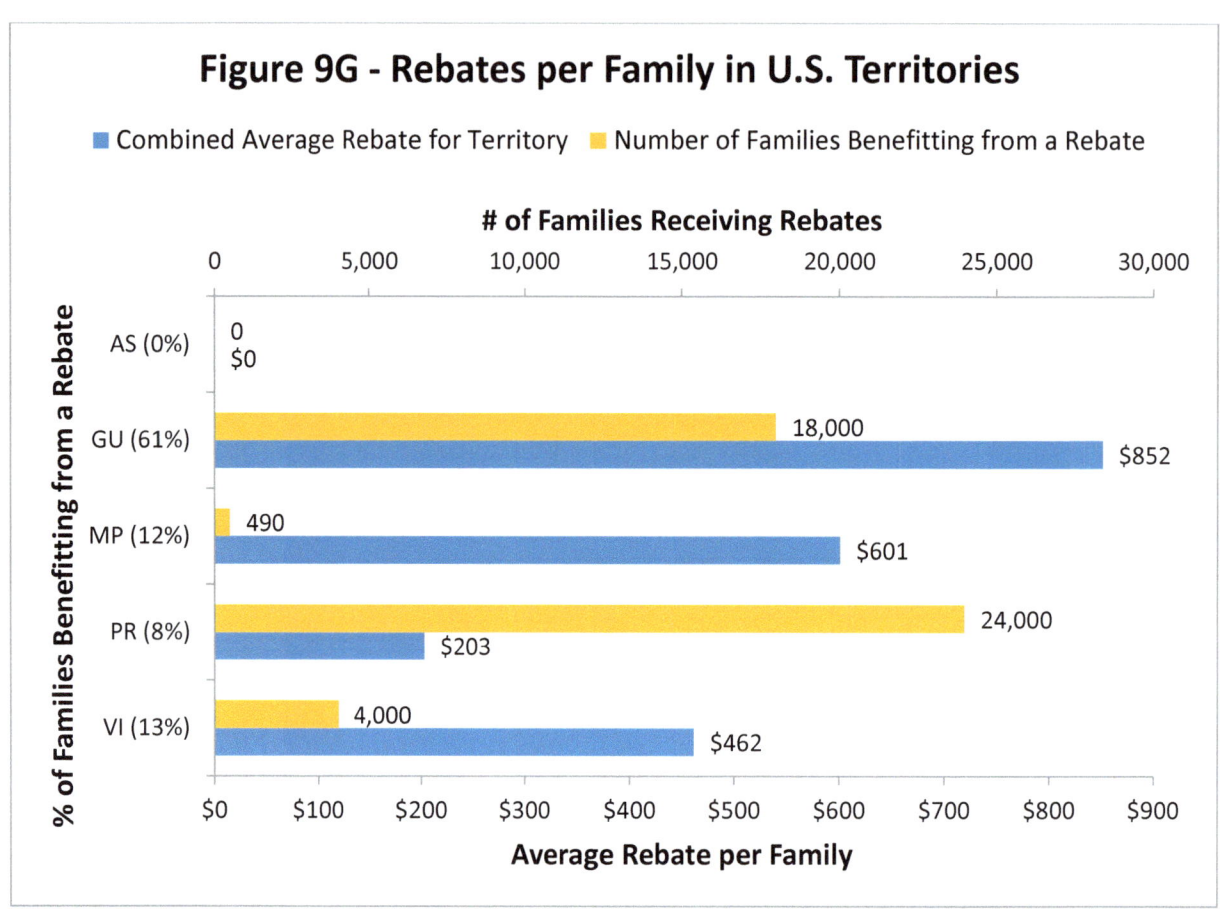

Figure 9G - Rebates per Family in U.S. Territories

In 2011, most health insurers met the required MLR standard and gave consumers the required value for their premiums. Approximately 90% of insurers in the individual market met the MLR standard. Approximately 89% met the standard in the small group market, and approximately 88% met the standard in the large group market. The average 2011 MLR for all insurance companies nationwide was approximately 84.3% in the individual market, 84.4% in the small group market, and 89.8% in the large group market. Actual MLRs varied widely among different insurance companies, with most MLRs between 72% and 98%.

The following chart (Figure 10) shows the distribution of enrollees within various MLR ranges for each market.

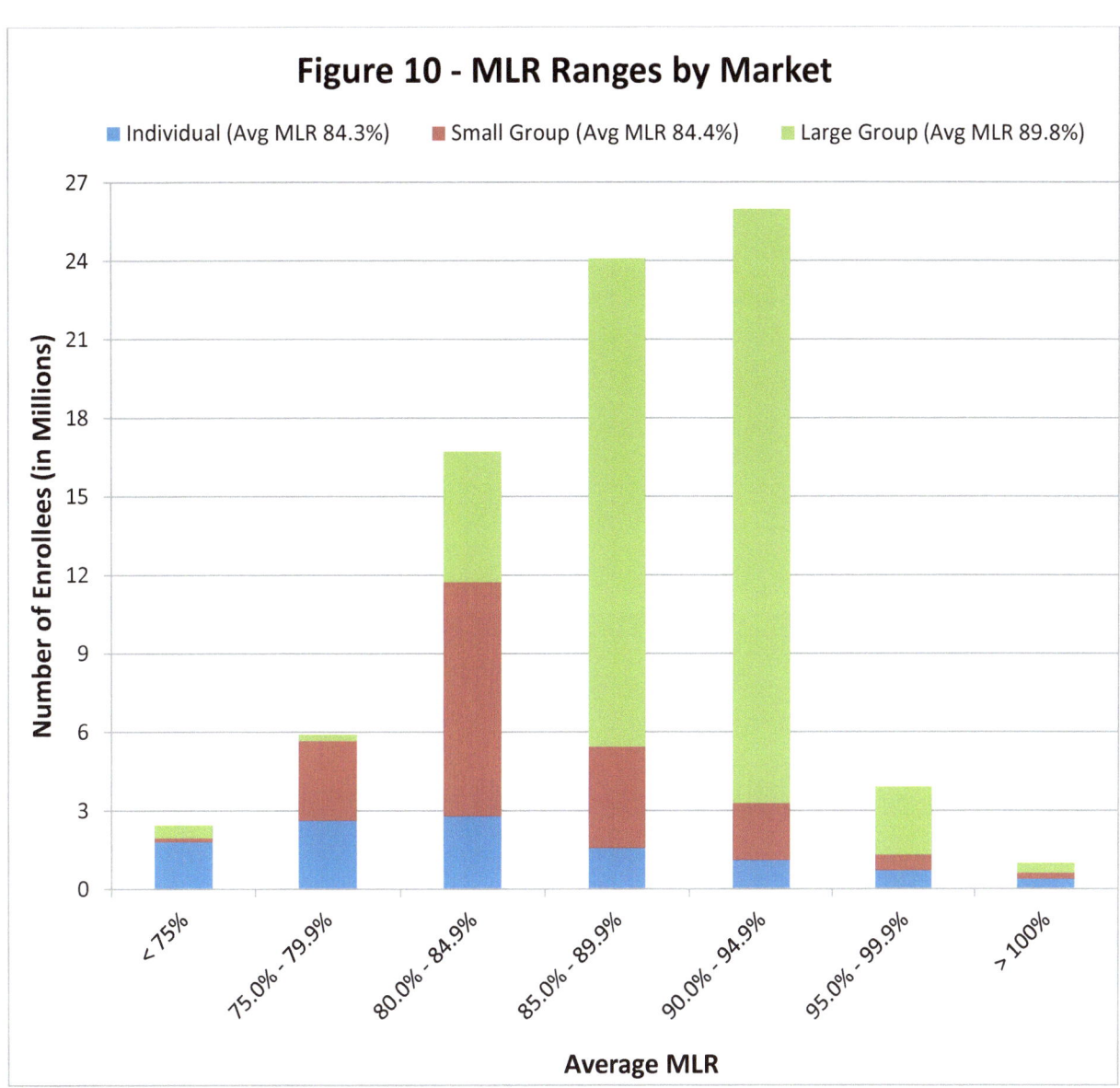

Figure 10 - MLR Ranges by Market

Conclusion

The 80/20 rule helps ensure that insurance companies provide consumers value for their premium dollars by making insurance companies spend premiums on patients' medical care rather than excessive administrative costs and profits. The rule discourages insurance companies from raising premium rates solely to increase profits since insurers must provide rebates if premium increases exceed increases in costs for medical services and improving quality of care. The 80/20 rule works in combination with other consumer protections in the Affordable Care Act, such as reviewing insurance companies' rates to ensure that premium increases are not unreasonable.

This report reflects health insurers' premium and spending in 2011, which was the first year for which insurers were required to report this information. Health insurers must report this information to HHS each year. We expect that this year and in the future, more and more insurers will provide the required value for health care premium dollars, especially since many insurers in the individual and small group markets will have to standardize their products to cover essential health benefits beginning in 2014, and that consumers will continue to benefit from the increased transparency the 80/20 rule provides.